SUDDEN DEATH

WAYNE SUTTON

Copyright 2020

This book is not intended as a substitute for the medical advice of physicians. The reader should regularly consult a physician in matters relating to his/her health, and particularly with respect to any symptoms that may require diagnosis or medical attention.

Although the publisher and the author have made every effort to ensure that the information in this book was correct at press time and while this publication is designed to provide accurate information in regard to the subject matter covered, the publisher and the author assume no responsibility for errors, inaccuracies, omissions, or any other inconsistencies herein and hereby disclaim any liability to any party for any loss, damage, or disruption caused by errors or omissions, whether such errors or omissions result from negligence, accident, or any other cause.

This publication is meant as a source of valuable information for the reader, however it is not meant as a substitute for direct expert assistance. If such level of assistance is required, the services of a competent professional should be sought.

Chapter One

Fear in your father's eyes is not an image you want to see. And it's one you will never forget.

I remember seeing my Dad lying on the table waiting to go into surgery, IV's in his arm and a truly scared look on his face.

Walking into the cold hallway to enter the surgery room, I saw tears in my stepmother's eyes. I whispered a prayer under my breath for my father as they carted him away under the bright fluorescent lights.

Forty-five years old. Quadruple bypass. My dad was scared. I was scared.

I wondered - what if? What if he didn't make it back through those cold double doors?

My dad made it back through the doors of the surgery room. Yet, he never fully recovered physically or financially. Ultimately, he lost his business, his hope, and his dignity because of this sickness. He couldn't keep up with the customers who needed his services, and even after several years he never really fully recovered.

I was also faced with the reality that my grandfather had died at fifty years old from a stroke. Also, my other grandfather had died in his fifties from a stroke after living years in a nursing home unable to take care of himself.

At this time, I was in my mid-twenties. Even though I was young, I began thinking of how heart disease could affect me one day.

Is heart disease truly something that just happens when you get older?

Now, I thought about getting older at times, but I didn't pay a lot of attention to it until a few years later when I had extremely high blood pressure. I was fighting headaches from hypertension and was starting to question my own future.

There must be a way to stop people from falling victim to heart disease.

For many people, heart disease is a battle they've fought for years. They have taken several medicines, had surgeries, stints, and stress tests repeatedly until finally, heart disease wins and the person simply dies.

I'll continue my story about my father in just a moment, but I want to share another story with you really quickly.

His name is unknown to me, yet I saw him lying lifeless upon the concrete sidewalk. While talking with a friend of mine, he simply stopped in a blink of an eye and fell backward to his death. His head landed upon the concrete so hard blood splattered. That incident reminded us of the precious life that had just been lost.

Call 911.

Call 911, now!

All I knew to do was pray and ask God for a miracle. I was praying, only releasing my hands from his body long enough for the EMT to attempt to "shock him" back to life. Sixty years old, instant, massive heart attack—in mere seconds he was dead.

Sudden death takes a toll when you are the observer. You recognize just how important your heart is. You also realize how deadly heart disease is.

I watched his wife sobbing over his corpse and again thought to myself there has to be a solution.

The ambulance took his body to the hospital. His wife sat beside him in the back of the ambulance, knowing she had spoken her last words to her husband.

Heart disease is a killer... often without warning.

The only purpose of heart disease is to destroy your life and kill you. Sometimes it's sudden, sometimes not so sudden—but the outcome, the final verdict is always the same—death.

My dad made it through open heart surgery. He came back through the double doors. However, because of the sickness and the circulation problems, he developed other issues including financial devastation.

Even throughout the bypass surgery, he had circulatory problems in other parts of his body. His life was far less than ideal. Heart disease caused him to live a poor quality of life.

Perhaps like me, you are beginning to recognize heart disease is an important subject that must be addressed. Sudden death occurs every day. Just as the man lying on the sidewalk, thousands upon thousands of people die every day. Thousands upon thousands are having their chests opened up for bypass surgery. Some make it out alive. Yet, some never do.

I was convinced there was a solution. This persuasion motivated me to spend time in prayer and seek the divine for a solution. I remember the prayer because I said it more than once. "God, there must be an answer. God, there has to be an answer to heart disease. I need you to reveal it to me."

I wasn't happy. I wasn't satisfied. I would not accept a "medicine only" cure or that I should eat better and exercise more. That all sounded great, but the sixty-year-old who suddenly fell dead was an athlete himself.

As you read this book, I want you to think about the people in your life. Maybe it's the man or woman in the mirror who has heart disease or is concerned about heart disease and circulatory issues.

I want you to think about that person. If it's you, take all the time you need to consider, "Is there a solution for me? Is there something I can do to change my life?"

Sudden death happens all too often because of heart disease. That's true! But God heard my prayer! I believe He heard yours too! I believe that God has brought this solution I'm about to reveal in this book to you. I am confident as you open up your mind and look closely at the material I will release, you will discover this as well.

I invite you to come to the truth that sudden death and heart disease can be a thing of the past. Am I talking a miracle here? Absolutely. Am I making a very bold statement? Absolutely.

The secret that has helped so many people—and I believe will help you change your life—is found in the next few pages of this book.

Enjoy the read…

Chapter Two

Sudden death is not always sudden. However, death is always death and often feels sudden. Heart disease is the number one cause of death in both men and women in the United States, claiming approximately one million lives annually.

One million!

Every thirty-three seconds, someone in the United States dies from cardiovascular disease. Every thirty-three seconds—the time it took you to read the fact above—somebody dies. That's equivalent to a September 11th-like tragedy repeating itself every twenty-four hours, three hundred and sixty-five days a year.

More people die of heart disease than HIV and *all* types of cancer combined. In fact, heart disease is the leading cause of death throughout the world. This year alone, more than nine hundred and twenty thousand Americans will suffer a heart attack! Nearly half of them, and this is very important, will occur without symptoms or prior warning signs.

250,000 Americans die annually of sudden cardiac death! That is 680 people every single day. Half of the victims of sudden cardiac death are under the age of sixty-five. So approximately 340 people under age sixty-five will die today from heart disease!

It's estimated that 80 million Americans have one or more type of heart disease. Actually, right now, almost 8 million Americans who are alive have had a heart attack.

But it's not just men. Sudden death doesn't occur just for men. Women are dying from cardiovascular disease as well. In fact, women account for just <u>over half</u> of the total heart disease deaths in the United States each year, although many people continue to believe it's just a "man's disease."

Worldwide, 8.6 *million* women die from heart disease each year, accounting for 1/3 of all deaths for women. And now, 42% of women who have heart attacks die within one year. That's compared to 24% of men. So heart disease is extremely dangerous for women. In fact, for women under 50 years old, a heart attack is twice as likely to be fatal compared to a man.

This is terrifying.

In America today, 8 million women are currently living with heart disease. And 350,000 of those women are under the age of 65.

430,000 American women have heart attacks every single year. If that's not startling enough—83,000 of these women are under the age of 65 and 35,000 are under the age of 55!

Sudden death is real.

267,000 women die each year from heart attacks. This is 600% more than those who die from breast cancer! I believe in cancer awareness. But I also believe it's time to look at heart disease and fight back with everything we have!

Sudden death occurs but a slow death is still sudden.

I was there when my father passed away. I literally caught his body and held him as he gasped for his last breath. When you're holding your dying father in your hands, your life changes. At that moment and from that moment, everything takes a different perspective.

I felt compassion as I held a lifeless body in my arms. It gave me the indignation to go against disease, to fight heart disease, and to rescue others. I want people to have the quality of life they deserve!

Slow death is still sudden.

For my father, slow death was the 10-12 years he fought. He battled from the time he recognized he had heart disease and other heart disease-related issues until his last breath in my arms.

I knew there had to be a solution.

Slow death may look slow, but it was painful for him. He lost his dignity and sense of honor. His life became a downward slope into a place of death. But even though we knew it was coming, the death was still sudden. I will always remember the moment his heart stopped, and he took his last breath.

Maybe you are thinking, "Well, I've not had a heart attack" or "I'm on medicine and my heart's okay… my blood pressure is okay." That's fine. But there is a better way.

One day, we will all face death. Until that time, you need to have a quality of life you can be excited about and enjoy. You must enjoy the adventures and people you have been blessed with. You need to have a truly good quality of life instead of taking pills, doing stress tests, and saying, "I can't do that. I can't hold out for that.

My energy level isn't what it used to be." Again, you need a good quality of life rather than sudden death that comes from years of suffering.

Slow death is still sudden.

Our family knew my father was sick. His friends knew he was sick; yet, it was still sudden when he died. The phone calls to family members and friends, as well as holding your dad's body in your arms as he passes away—slow death is still sudden death.

This chapter is a gift to you. As you're reading this and thinking about your own heart and heartbeat, this book is for you.

As you think about the people who are important to you, those whose lives you could possibly extend and improve, give them a copy of this book. Let them know it is a gift, and they can all avoid sudden cardiac death.

Chapter Three

I have seen death, and I have experienced life. I choose life!

I prayed. And I began to seek a solution. I was determined to witness the cycle of sickness and early death in my family end once and for all.

My seeking included asking those in the medical field lots of questions (which left me discouraged many times), searching the infamous Google what seemed like a million times and of course, buying the health and wellness books from the local bookstore.

I read, examined, and found so many half-answers, myths, outright lies, and false information. In fact, it all sounded the same after a while. Eat better; eat differently; exercise more, and then of course, if needed—swallow a mouthful of pills with a long list of potentially deadly side-effects.

Discover the truth in this book most people and a gross majority of medical professionals are either ignorant of or simply do not care to know! More pills. That's their answer.

Prescription medicines may help deal with the onset of heart disease or manage it for a while, but they will not reverse it. Period. Now, I am not a doctor, but I urge you to ask *any* doctor, and they will very confidently tell you I am 100% correct.

There is a solution!

A single phone call from someone who also honored life changed my life forever. It's the reason you are reading this book today.

I was driving over to my favorite lunch spot, with my soul set on eating delicious chicken fajitas when my thoughts and entire day were interrupted and my life perpetually transformed.

"Wayne, I found it," he spoke with absolute clarity. "I found the solution for heart disease."

He held my attention.

"This is science. It's proven by clinical studies, and it's available today—"

He attempted to continue but I interrupted him instead.

Have you ever truly prayed for something, hoped one day it would show up in your life, yet, had no idea when or if it would?

That call was the solution for me.

"I want to hear more," I replied. "If this is real, we have to tell everyone about—"

"It is real! There is absolute proof, and it is 100% guaranteed." Science. Proven. 100% Guaranteed.

OK, full attention.

I discovered over the next few hours of phone calls and my own research that what I had prayed about for years was finally available. It was truly even a greater answer than I had imagined. The answer was simple yet powerful.

Before I share the cause and correction I discovered, allow me to ask you a few questions. Do you or anyone you know have any of the following health struggles?

- Heart disease

- Diabetes

- High blood pressure

- Chronic pain

- Arthritis

- Erectile dysfunction

- Alzheimer's

- Depression

- Migraine headaches

- Kidney issues

- Dementia

- Multiple Sclerosis

- Menopause

- Cold hands or feet

- Lack of energy

What is interesting is that everyone with these issues shares one thing in common—they *all* lack nitric oxide (NO). The lack of nitric oxide causes your blood vessels to become stiff and sticky, almost like Velcro.

Why does this matter? Because as this happens, plaque forms and sticks to the walls of your blood vessels. Over time, it blocks your blood flow. Consequently, your entire body is damaged!

So what is nitric oxide?

Many people think it's the "laughing gas" at the dentist's office. Some people think it's the fuel for race cars. But it's neither.

Nitric oxide is actually a molecule our bodies produce to assist the 50 trillion cells to communicate with each other throughout the entire body.

Nitric oxide is a miracle! And it is very important in the following cellular activities:

- Help memory and behavior by transmitting information between nerve cells in the brain

- Assist the immune system in fighting off bacteria and defending against tumors!

- Regulate blood pressure by dilating arteries.

- Reduce inflammation

- Improve your sleep quality

- Increase your recognition of smell

- Increase both endurance and strength

Over 60,000 studies have been conducted on nitric oxide in the last 20 years—over 60 thousand studies! Furthermore, in 1998 the Nobel Prize for medicine was awarded for the discovery of the signaling role of nitric oxide. This is a *huge* advancement in your life!

Bye-bye heart disease.

Nitric oxide has received the most attention due to its cardiovascular benefits. That's why you are reading this book.

Allow me to take you on a brief, eye-opening journey of how this powerful miracle is your miracle and how to *amplify it to save your life!* Bold? Yep, enjoy as we journey a little deeper.

Nitric oxide has received the most attention due to its powerful cardiovascular benefits. It works perfectly within the body.

The interior surface of our arteries (endothelium) produces nitric oxide because our bodies were designed to bring healing. That's the good news. The bad news, however, is that once plaque builds up in your arteries (atherosclerosis), it greatly reduces the ability of the arteries to produce the life-giving nitric oxide.

When your arteries can produce adequate levels of nitric oxide, it increases blood flow, prevents fatty deposits from sticking to blood vessel walls, keeps the walls from getting thick and stiff, and prevents arteries from narrowing.

One of the first researchers to study the roles of nitric oxide in cardiovascular health stated that when the endothelium is healthy it's like Teflon and things don't stick. However, when it's unhealthy—as in most people today—it is more like Velcro in your body!

What damages the endothelium?

Life. In fact, all of the major culprits in heart disease: being overweight, unhealthy diet, smoking, sleep apnea, high blood pressure, high levels of homocysteine and lipoprotein all damage the endothelium. Sadly, a damaged endothelium will not produce enough nitric oxide, which results in more damage to the endothelium. Thus, the downward cycle continues.

Doesn't heart disease require prescription medicine or surgery?

Not always. Now, I am not a doctor or cardiologist. However, I am a seeker of truth and the truth has set me free! Using the solution you are about to discover in this booklet, I have totally broken free from the fear and even the reality of heart disease. Let me also state that I am neither an exercise junky nor am I an "organic only" food connoisseur.

I am for *all* of the above, but they are not for me. So why do I feel so passionate about this?

It works.

This program has *tons* of scientific data to back up my claims. Plus, we have *thousands* of people who have overcome and are now living healthy!

Before you find yourself too excited about this book, I want to share an important fact: the main product that releases nitric oxide is arginine. It's a miracle but there's a catch.

All arginine is not the same and how you choose the proper arginine supplement will determine your results. I decided to find and use the very best because my life depends on it! And so does yours.

First, running to the local vitamin store and grabbing arginine supplements is not the right answer. In fact, it could hurt you more than it could help you. Why? Arginine has a very short half- life of about 75 minutes or so. Also, synthetic arginine may cause gastrointestinal distress. So unless you want to take small doses every single hour or two every day, you need a better solution.

Yes, there are different forms of arginine. You must take the proper form, along with the right amount of citrulline, which is another important amino acid and a major factor in helping the body produce nitric oxide.

Citrulline also helps extend the half-life of arginine, and itself is converted into nitric oxide. Supplementing with citrulline is very important as part of your regimen.

The Key?

Before I release the key to overcoming heart disease to you, let me share a few other important supplements I have uncovered. Now, before you find yourself too excited—and believe me; you can easily do so once you see the full power of this system—take a quick look at the other supplements.

Vitamin C

When I first began my search for supplementation, I found the power behind good ol' vitamin C. Although vitamin C is very common, the knowledge of what it has for our health has not been that well-known—until recently…

Researchers at the University of California stated that participants who consumed approximately 500 milligrams of vitamin C supplement per day saw a 24% reduction in plasma C-reactive protein (CPR) levels after only 2 months.

What does that mean for you?

C-reactive protein is a marker of inflammation. Evidence is showing that chronic inflammation is linked to an increase in heart disease, diabetes, cancer, arthritis, and even Alzheimer's disease.

This is really important. Dr. James Enstrom from the University of California studied the vitamin intake of over 11,000 people for 10 years. His findings? He found that 300 mg of vitamin C a day reduced the risk of heart disease by more than 50% in men and 40% in women.

Doctor G.C. Willis found that people taking 1,500 mg of vitamin C a day for 12 months actually reversed plaque, while those who didn't take vitamin C had worsening plaque. It's very clear that vitamin C is necessary for vascular health.

Vitamin D

While you are out catching some rays this summer, think about vitamin D. Often called the "sunshine vitamin," it is produced in your skin in response to sunlight.

Vitamin D is a fat-soluble vitamin in a family of compounds that includes vitamins D1, D2, and D3, and can affect as many as 2,000 genes in the body. So what are the functions of vitamin D in your life? Perhaps the most vital is regulating the absorption of calcium and phosphorus, and the facilitation of normal immune system function.

A sufficient amount of vitamin D is important for normal growth and the development of limbs and teeth, as well as improved resistance against certain diseases.

In the largest study of its kind to evaluate the relationship between vitamin D levels and coronary heart disease, vitamin D deficiency was observed in 70.4% of patients undergoing coronary angiography—an imaging test used to see blood flows through the arteries in the heart.

Vitamin D deficiency was associated with a higher prevalence of coronary disease, with a 32% higher occurrence in patients with the lowest vitamin D levels and a near 20% higher frequency of severe disease affecting multiple vessels. A progressive increase in heart disease was found according to the severity of vitamin D deficiency.

Vitamin K2

It is time to finally unleash this hidden gem in the world of nutrition. Vitamin K2 supplementation is just beginning to receive the recognition it deserves, and you can benefit greatly from this once unknown supplement.

Vitamin K2 has several functions in the body that help us to use calcium efficiently by getting it to where the body needs it and out of the place it doesn't.

Dutch researchers discovered very strong links between the benefits of vitamin K2 intake with arterial calcification and cardiovascular death.

In fact, in a clinical trial of nearly 5,000 older Dutch men and women known as the Rotterdam study, participants with the highest consumption of vitamin K2 had a 50% reduction in arterial calcification and death from cardiovascular disease, as well as a 25% decline in overall mortality.

Are you getting excited yet? Continue on…

Grape Skin and Seed Extracts

Grapes, along with their leaves and sap, have been traditional treatments in Europe for thousands of years. Grape seed extract is derived from the ground-up seed of red wine grapes.

There is very strong evidence that the extract is beneficial for many issues including poor circulation and high cholesterol. Full of antioxidants, grape skin extract may help prevent the formulation of unhealthful plaque in arteries, improve capillary resistance, and bonds with collagen to create more flexibility in the vessels and capillaries.

Also, *Medical News Today* reports that the extract can prevent age-related cognitive decline, speed up healing, and decrease swelling and inflammation.

So can grape extracts help you?

Yes!

In another study, volunteers were given a placebo or 200 and 400 mg dosages of grape seed extract for 12 weeks. The levels of oxidatively modified LDL levels (considered a possible marker for artery disease) from this given extract were significantly reduced compared to the placebo group.

Now, let me state again that I am not a doctor. So do your own research as well. Having said that, I witnessed the typical, medical procedures when it comes to cardiovascular disease, and I have seen the alternative. I choose the healthy way!

When the nurse whispers, and you become truly scared…

Blake suffered a stroke while at work and immediately found it impossible to stand on his own, speak, or beg for assistance.

Grunts were his words as his co-worker Cindy attempted to decipher his noises and frantic actions.

Stroke.

He was only 52 years old. However, he learned quickly that his circulatory issues were not taking the time to ask if he was ready or "old enough" to face this condition.

He was blessed to make it to the hospital in time for the blood clot to be treated, and he faced no permanent effects from the stroke. Yet, from the testing, they found up to 60% blockage in his arteries and were suggesting much more invasive treatment.

A few weeks later, someone introduced the information found in this book to Blake and his wife. His wife Peggy, a registered nurse, did her research and suggested he give it a try.

He had been using a product the author of this book suggested for about 4 months when he went back for a follow-up with his doctor. That's when he heard the technicians looking at the chart and whispering.

"Excuse me," he interrupted, "what's going on with my results?" He was nervous. Actually, Blake was absolutely scared. What had they found?

Waiting for the nurses to respond was terrifying and his fear showed.

"Please," he begged. "I've already had a stroke and waiting for these results is not helping my blood pressure." Anxious and very scared, he watched the nurses whisper and noticed their confusion.

"Mr. Cale, your results are not normal," she quietly said. "They are not ordinary."

No Hills - No Valleys!

The nurses and the doctor were amazed that in just a few short months, they could not detect the typical and measurable "hills and valleys" on their testing equipment. What did that mean?

No plaque.

This is why they were whispering. They could not understand how anyone at Blake's age and weight could have virtually zero plaque build-up. Furthermore, the fact that Blake had recently had a stroke, yet, now seemed to be a walking miracle, truly amazed the nurses and the doctor!

Read that again…

Blake went from up to 60% blockage to numbers so low they could not detect *any* on their diagnostic machines! He had perfect blood pressure and no blockages within just months of using the information in this book.

Seven years later, as of this writing, Blake reports a blood pressure of 105/65 without taking any blood pressure medicine. And, Blake has lost over 70 pounds with the help of this information. And yes, he is still free of blockages!

The Until Moment

Rome Batchelor from Wilson, NC is the friend of mine who called me that day and shared the information in this book. Like me, Rome was searching for the solution in his own life. He was suffering from headaches, fatigue, and then more stress as he was popping pills from the doctor and literally praying he didn't get a stroke or heart attack.

He had a number of "close calls" and episodes. He was certain he was on the brink of a heart attack. When he was fortunate enough to discover the solution, he called me and immediately started using this remedy himself.

Here are his exact words:

> The day my product arrived my blood pressure was running 171/117 and after just 45 minutes on the product it dropped to 155/88 and by the next morning, it was 120 over 77!
>
> That is perfect blood pressure which I have had issues with for over 25 years now since I was in the Army.
>
> After 5 days, my energy was up and my sleep was noticeably improved. Also for some odd reason, my knees have not been hurting even after walking an hour on concrete and they haven't hurt at all for weeks and the

only thing different is this product.

Also, I've noticed a huge increase in my ability to breathe clearly. Breathing easily has been an issue for me for decades and now I feel like running again!

I have cold Urticaria, which is an allergy to cold that causes an itching/burning rash on the back of my hands when I get cold. I have had it for about 10 years and even up to a few months ago. After 8 or so months on this product, it's not happening even after walking my dog in 29-degree weather! - Rome

Life saved. Life extended. Plus, the energy and vitality to enjoy life!

Your Solution — Your Answer

The pages you have read or, at least, skimmed over to this part of the book proves you are truly ready for an answer!

This is it!

In my search and prayers for an answer, I discovered that almost everyone had an "answer." Yet, no one could prove their theory. I was not about to risk my life on their theory or old wives' tales. I needed *the solution*.

So if you're ready to cut through the nonsense, hype, and years of research as you finally discover your answer—here it is.

I made a promise to myself once I found this solution. This book is that promise. What was the promise? I would never back down or be covert in my message. I will never apologize for my bluntness or be anything other than direct and to the point.

If you still have a heartbeat then you need this solution. What is this solution? I am glad you asked. It is a synergistic blend of scientifically proven supplements in the exact amounts that are very easy to consume every day.

Are you finding yourself excited yet?

Great!

The worst thing I could do for you is "beat around the bush," ask you to do more research, simply pick up a few supplements and hope you have the right synergistic blends. You are more important than that. Therefore, I am blatantly and boldly telling you to grab a hold of this solution and experience the truth of your new life!

Now, because you have read this far, you are obviously searching and seeking a healthy life. Imagine a supplement you can take once or twice a day that accomplishes all of the benefits you have read about in this book. What would that do for you?

How would you feel knowing you can literally wake up knowing that overnight, your body was producing nitric oxide, which allowed it to heal itself? And how would you feel knowing that as you go through your day, every moment, your body is producing the perfect amount of nitric oxide? Day after day, you are becoming healthier throughout your entire circulatory system!

Because you have read this far, and you are obviously seeking a healthy and long life, I am going to do everything in my power to help you.

Like me, the person who placed this book in your hands has dedicated his or her life to helping others walk in health and escape the fear of sudden death and heart disease.

That person is most likely not a doctor, neither am I. However, as medical researchers, we can share the facts and words from the doctors who are using this product and recommending it to their patients!

What's your next step?

Contact the person who gave you this book, and ask him or her for more information, as well as some samples of this amazing formula.

This product is not available on Amazon or at GNC, etc. It is available by referral from the person who shared this book with you.

So call or text the person at____and let him or her know you would like some more information.

Your heart will thank you!

Wayne Sutton

Get More Information Now From:

Other Unsolicited Testimonials

"When I saw how this product was helping my husband I was amazed. Because heart disease runs in my family, I decided to have a blood circulation test and was shocked to see that my blood circulation was at level 5. On a scale of 1 to 5 that is the worst! I haven't had any of the typical heart-related symptoms, so I thought I was okay. That's why they call it the "Silent Killer." After taking this product, I took the test again. I am pleased to say that my level was down to a 2. I couldn't be happier about that!

Both my husband and I love this product and will continue to take it forever!" ~ Judy

"I have heart disease, kidney (renal) failure and diabetes. I had my first heart attack when I was 31 years old. I had the bypass surgery and all the stuff they did back in the 1970s. I had five more heart attacks over the years and by 1993, only 25% of my heart was working.

I had a heart transplant, which was a success, but I had to take mega, mega drugs. I was on 36 different drugs a day but now, because of this product, I'm only on about 4 or 5. Two years ago, I was diagnosed with renal failure. I was getting prepared to be on dialysis when I was introduced to this product. After taking it for about 3 weeks, I went in for a blood test for my kidneys and the doctor said, 'it looks like you don't have to start dialysis; let's put it off and see what happens.'

We waited and more blood tests showed my kidneys were improving. The doctor had been considering putting me on a kidney transplant list, and three months later he said he didn't need to do that. I was taking 8 shots of insulin a day because of my diabetes. After starting this product, I was down to 2 a day and now, I'm not on any insulin shots. This product has changed my health and my life!" ~ Larry

"I have severe crippling rheumatoid arthritis, which was so bad that last year I had to quit my job as a Youth Pastor and volunteer for Young Life. When I was introduced to this product five months ago, along with my arthritis, I was having some heart problems, which is hereditary in my family. My blood pressure went soaring and I was having pains in my chest and down my arm. I was having trouble breathing and I couldn't swallow. My friend started me on this product and within 3 days, the pain in my chest had subsided, and I was starting to breathe better. And the phenomenal thing was I woke up in the morning and the pain in my hands was gone!

Within a month, I was pain-free. I also had cysts inside my thighs; they are gone. I had restless leg syndrome. I don't have that anymore. I had muscle cramps in my legs so that when I lay down at night the pain would tear me apart, and I couldn't sleep. I had acid reflux, and it is all gone. I've had bouts of pleurisy since I was a little girl and haven't had any since starting this product. My lungs are healthy and my blood pressure is down where it should be. I feel like I'm twenty years old again.

I'm back to the Youth Ministry and I'm back with Young Life. There are so many things that have changed in my life. I feel like I have a whole new life and I'm starting over!" ~ Sherry

"I suffered from pain and chronic fatigue throughout my whole life. About three years ago, I was diagnosed with fibromyalgia and chronic fatigue syndrome. My good friend's family sent me some of this product and their only request was for me to get better.

And I have! I wasn't able to get out of bed and walk. Within three months, I was able to get right up out of bed and function throughout the day. I get very emotional just thinking about how the product has changed my life!" ~ Dawn

"I've been dealing with high blood pressure since I was 22 years old. I used to manage it with exercise and diet, but it got progressively worse over the years. By the time I was 30, I was sent home from work because my boss was so concerned about me due to stress, high blood pressure, high cholesterol, even though I was taking medication. By the time I was 37 years old, I had a heart attack. My blood pressure was 280/260. Since then, I've been in the hospital numerous times. I've spent thousands of dollars researching to see if I could find something to help me lower my blood pressure naturally.

A friend sent me information about this product. The first time I took it, within 35 minutes I felt different. That evening, my blood pressure was down to 135/96, and I had not taken any blood pressure pills that evening. I was amazed. The next morning, my blood pressure was 128/92. Within 3 days, I decided to stop taking my blood pressure pills and haven't taken any since! Now my blood pressure runs about 119/77 each day (without any blood pressure pills). It's unbelievable! This product has changed my life!" ~ Gary

"Fourteen months ago, I was an absolute disaster. You could probably measure my life expectancy in a matter of months, if not weeks. My blood pressure was out of control; my diabetes was out of control. I was having problems with my brain because of diabetes, and also having problems with my bladder, my kidneys, you name it. I couldn't walk more than a couple of hundred yards without resting.

I heard about this from a friend and started taking about six scoops a day. The first thing I noticed was I could walk further and further distances. I noticed that my overall health was improving rapidly. I was on 17 prescriptions, taking about 40 pills a day. That's about 1200 pills a month, over 14,000 pills a year. I knew I was not going to live long in this world.

This product made it possible for me to get off almost all of those pills! I am totally off eleven of the 17 prescriptions and the other six, I'm taking in reduced amounts. My insulin intake has gone from 154 units to just a fraction. As a matter of fact, I just got a letter in the mail today saying, "Take one shot of Lantus at night, 24 units." That is amazing! I now look forward to the future, and I feel great!" ~ Mike

"I started taking this product and my high liver enzymes, which were off the chart went back to normal. My triglycerides went from about 900 to 200. My blood pressure dropped from 157/92 to 122/78. My sexual function improved. I lost 30 pounds, and I have more energy than I've had in a long, long time." ~ Dan

"My husband is 80 years old. He started this product around the first part of June 2013. We decided to try this product as his heart had gotten quite bad. He was spending more time lying on the couch than being up. He was exhausted most of the time. We had planned a spring trip to go to Washington & Idaho to ride bicycles trails but decided that there was no way we could go. The drive alone would have exhausted him.

God's timing is perfect.

Around that time, a friend told us about this product. We had an appointment with Bob's heart doctor. We told our doctor about the product. He watched the video and said it looked good to him. Especially since there wasn't any more he could do for him. He said go ahead and try it.

Bob was on the product just a little over a week and could feel the change. He was taking 4 scoops a day. To make a long story short, after about a month-and-a-half, we decided to go on our vacation. He did wonderful. We rode bikes all over Idaho and Washington. On one ride, we actually went 18 miles. There is no way we could have done this if the Lord had not brought this product into our lives. He has now been on the product for 3 months and is doing good. He is now taking 3 scoops a day. I thank the Lord every day that I have my husband back." ~ Carol

Contact the person who gave you this book, and ask him or her for more information and some samples of our amazing supplement.

Now, it's not available on Amazon or at GNC, etc. It's available by referral from the person who shared this book with you.

So, call or text the person at____and let him or her know you would like some more information.

Your heart will thank you!
Wayne Sutton

Get More Information Now From:

*To order copies of this book go to www.OrderTeamBooks.com or call the office at 910-233-2511.

This book is not intended as a substitute for the medical advice of physicians. The reader should regularly consult a physician in matters relating to his/her health, and particularly with respect to any symptoms that may require diagnosis or medical attention.

Made in the USA
Middletown, DE
17 March 2021